COMPLETE GUIDE TO CHINESE PULSE DIAGNOSIS

A Comprehensive Guide To Pulse Assessment For Health

TONY MICHAEL

Contents

CHAPTER ONE
Chinese Pulse Diagnosis: An Overview

Traditional Chinese medicine practitioners employ a method called "Chinese pulse diagnosis" to evaluate a patient's health by monitoring subtle changes in the rhythm of their pulse. It has been used for hundreds of years and is still commonly used today as part of traditional Chinese medicine (TCM).

One's pulse can provide insight into the health of one's internal organs, meridian pathways, and energy flow as a whole. The strength, quality, rhythm, and other features of the pulse can provide vital information to a qualified practitioner about a patient's health as they palpate the pulse at various pulse locations on the body.

Interpreting the pulse in Chinese medicine is a complicated process that takes into account a wide range of variables, including the pulse's rate, width, intensity, and quality.

These traits can provide information about a person's constitution, general health, and any underlying health issues or imbalances.

Different pulse sites on the radial artery of both wrists are frequently checked, as they are linked to various TCM organs and meridians.

The practitioner palpates the pulse with their fingertips, using varying amounts of pressure and paying close attention to the intricacies in the features of the pulse.

Pulse diagnosis in Chinese medicine is a complex and intricate practice that experts say takes years to master. As part of a more thorough evaluation of the patient's health, TCM practitioners will also use observation, questioning, and examination of the tongue and other physical indications.

In Chinese medicine, a patient's pulse can be used to gain insight into their overall health and influence treatment options. Examination of the pulse is used to diagnose underlying health problems and create a treatment plan that may include acupuncture, herbal medicine, dietary changes, and other methods.

Diagnostic Pulse Theory And Practice

The practice of Chinese pulse diagnosis is grounded in a number of core concepts and beliefs of TCM.

Among these are:

• In TCM, Qi (vital energy) and Blood are viewed as the primary substances that permeate and nourish the many organs and tissues of the body.

The pulse is thought to reveal the state of the body's Qi and Blood in terms of quantity, quality, and circulation. A trained pulse diagnostician can determine the health of a patient's Qi and Blood by observing its strength, depth, and rhythm.

• Yin and Yang are fundamental notions in TCM. They reflect opposite yet complementary energies in nature. Evaluation of the pulse for Yin and Yang imbalances is central to the practice of pulse diagnostics.

A slow and feeble pulse, for instance, could point to a Yang shortage, while a strong and quick one could indicate an excess of Yang. The Yin and Yang balance in a patient's body can be determined through pulse diagnostics by a skilled practitioner.

• Each organ has an associated meridian or channel through which Qi flows in traditional Chinese medicine.

It is thought that the health of various organs and meridians can be gauged by feeling the pulse at specific locations on the body.

The radial artery pulse, for instance, might indicate the health of the heart, liver, kidneys, lungs, and spleen, among other organs. A practitioner can learn about the condition of the associated organs and meridians by palpating the pulse at these sites.

• Another important concept in TCM is the Five Element Theory, which provides a comprehensive account of the complex and ever-changing interactions between the body's various systems.

A person's pulse can reveal whether or not their body is in harmony with the five elements of wood, fire, earth, metal, and water. For instance, the Liver and Gallbladder are connected to the Wood element, therefore an abnormally fast or slow pulse rate could indicate an imbalance there.

• Assessing the depth, rate, width, strength, and rhythm of the pulse are all important factors in Chinese pulse diagnosis. The characteristics of a patient's pulse are said to reveal information about the health of a patient's organs, meridians, and substances. Dampness is indicated by a floaty, smooth pulse, while Liver Qi stagnation is indicated by a wiry, choppy pulse.

Overall, Chinese pulse diagnosis is a complicated and nuanced procedure that calls for a thorough familiarity with TCM principles and theories, as well as significant clinical experience.

In TCM, it is used to evaluate a patient's health and direct treatment decisions with the goal of achieving a state of equilibrium and optimal health.

CHAPTER TWO
Traditional Chinese Medicine (TCM) Places A Premium On The Use Of Pulse Analysis

Several factors contribute to the significance of pulse diagnosis in traditional Chinese medicine (TCM):

• TCM practitioners can obtain a plethora of information about a patient's health condition in a non-invasive manner through pulse diagnostic.

An experienced practitioner can determine the health of a patient's Qi, Blood, Yin, Yang, organs, meridians, and other systems by carefully palpating the pulse at different pulse sites. The results of this test can be combined with those of other diagnostic approaches, such as patient observation and inquiry, to form a more complete picture of the patient's health.

• Traditional Chinese Medicine places a premium on tailoring each patient's care to their specific needs. Practitioners can better meet the individual needs of their patients with the aid of pulse diagnostics.

A practitioner can learn about the patient's underlying imbalances or patterns of disharmony in the body by listening to the patient's pulse and analyzing its unique qualities. This tailored approach to care has the potential to improve efficiency and precision.

• Pulse diagnostics can pick up on even the most subtle of imbalances in the body long before any outward symptoms appear. It can aid in the early detection of patterns of disharmony, allowing for the implementation of preventative interventions prior to the deterioration of a health condition.

TCM's emphasis on resolving underlying causes of illness is consistent with this preventative strategy.

• Pulse diagnosis is utilized not only for the first evaluation, but also for keeping tabs on how well a patient is responding to treatment. By monitoring changes in the patient's pulse characteristics over the course of treatment, a practitioner can gain important insight into the treatment's efficacy. The treatment plan can then be modified as necessary to achieve the best possible outcomes.

• Pulse diagnosis is consistent with the holistic perspective of traditional Chinese medicine, which sees the body as a whole. It provides a complete picture of the patient's health by allowing doctors to evaluate the interplay between the patient's organs, meridians, and substances. Treatment techniques, such as herbal medication, acupuncture, dietary suggestions, and lifestyle changes, that address the underlying imbalances can be selected with the help of this thorough diagnosis.

• The patient-practitioner interaction in TCM is heavily reliant on accurate pulse diagnosis. Patient involvement in the diagnostic procedure is enhanced by the tactile nature of pulse diagnosis, which can also foster a sense of trust, connection, and communication between the practitioner and patient. In TCM, this connection is seen as crucial since it improves our comprehension of the patient's situation and opens up new avenues for treatment.

TCM's pulse diagnosis is a fundamental and valuable diagnostic tool because it allows for a holistic assessment of a patient's health condition, guides individualized treatment, aids in the early detection of imbalances, monitors the progress of treatment, promotes a holistic understanding of the body, and fosters a strong patient-practitioner relationship.

Pulse Point Locations

Several spots on the inner side of the wrist, specifically along the radial artery, are used in TCM to feel the patient's pulse. Different organs and meridian pathways are linked to these specific pulse spots. Primary acupoints for TCM pulse diagnosis are:

• Cun (Inch) – Positioned on the radial artery at the same level as the thumb, nearest to the hand.

• Guan (Pass) is between the Cun and Chi pulse points on the radial artery.

• Chi (Cubit) – Level with the tip of the little finger on the radial artery, just below the elbow.

The "Three Cun" refer to the most prevalent pulse sites utilized in Traditional Chinese Medicine (TCM) pulse diagnosis: The Cun, Guan, and Chi. The following are their corresponding bodily organs and meridian pathways:

• The status of the lungs is reflected in the cun (inch) reading, which also reveals details on the health of the skin and the large intestine.

• The state of the Spleen is reflected in the Guan (Pass), which also reveals information about the Liver and the health of the muscles.

• Chi (Cubit) reflects the state of the Kidney and gives insight into the health of the Heart and vascular system as a whole.

Depending on their training and experience, TCM practitioners may also employ pulse sites other than the Three Cun in pulse diagnosis.

Bilateral Jing-Well points, Ying-Spring points, Shu-Stream points, and Luo-Connecting points are also important pulse sites that are linked to particular meridian pathways and internal organs.

Pulse diagnosis is a crucial part of Traditional Chinese Medicine, but it is a very delicate and difficult technique that can only be properly understood through years of practice. Treatment decisions are made after a thorough evaluation of the location, quality, depth, and other aspects of the pulse that reveal the underlying patterns of disharmony in the body.

CHAPTER THREE
Methods Relying On Palpation

Practitioners of traditional Chinese medicine (TCM) take a patient's pulse by palpating specific locations along the radial artery.

To learn more about the pulse's features and characteristics, various pressures and manipulations are used in these methods. In TCM, diagnosing the pulse often involves palpation, and some of the most popular methods are:

• To feel the pulse beneath the skin's surface, press your fingertips gently upon the pulse point. The practitioner's goal and the patient's condition will determine how much pressure is used. By applying pressure, a medical professional can evaluate the pulse's depth, width, and overall strength.

• Feel for a pulse that is "floating" or "superficial" under the fingertips, also known as "floating." Conditions of external or Yang excess, such as fever or acute illness, may be indicated by a pulse that seems to float.

• Feeling for a "sinking" or "deep" pulse under the fingertips is what we mean when we talk about sinking. Conditions of inner or Yin excess, such as cold or chronic illness, may be indicated by a sagging pulse.

• Sliding: This entails making a sliding motion with the fingertips along the pulse point to evaluate its smoothness or roughness. A healthy smooth pulse may imply no discord or blockage in the meridians, while a rough pulse may indicate the opposite.

• By rotating the fingertips in a circular motion over the pulse site, the quality of the pulse may be evaluated from multiple angles. If the pulse pattern is altered in any way, rolling can assist reveal it.

• TCM pulse diagnosis also makes use of other palpation techniques, such as identifying whether the pulse is "wiry" (similar to the sensation of a taut wire), "slippery" (similar to the sensation of slipping or smoothness), "choppy" (similar to the sensation of an uneven or interrupted pulse), or "hollow" (similar to the sensation of a weak or empty pulse). These methods can reveal more details regarding the pulse's characteristics.

Pulse diagnosis in TCM relies heavily on palpation procedures, which take a great deal of ability, sensitivity, and experience in order to correctly evaluate the qualities and patterns of disharmony in the patient's pulse. Pulse palpation is used as one piece of a larger diagnostic puzzle that takes into account the rate, rhythm, strength, depth, width, and other qualitative properties of the pulse as well as results from other diagnostic tests.

Analysis Of Pulse Characteristics (Such As Rate, Rhythm, Width, And Intensity)

Traditional Chinese medicine (TCM) pulse diagnosis entails analyzing the pulse's depth, pace, rhythm, width, and intensity in order to deduce the source of any imbalances felt by the patient. These pulse properties are seen as significant indications of the health of the organs and meridians, and can aid in the development of effective therapeutic plans.

In Traditional Chinese Medicine (TCM), pulse diagnosis is based on the following properties of the patient's pulse:

• The depth of the pulse is the distance from the fingertips to the heart. Depending on their intensity, TCM classifies pulses as either "floating" (superficial), "normal," or "sinking" (deep). Conditions of external or Yang excess, such as fever or acute illness, may be indicated by a pulse that seems to float.

Conditions of inner or Yin excess, such as cold or chronic illness, may be indicated by a sagging pulse. A healthy pulse is defined as one that is of a normal depth.

• Pulse rate indicates how quickly or slowly the heart is pumping blood throughout the body. Pulses are categorized as slow, normal, or rapid in Traditional Chinese Medicine. If your pulse is slow, it could be because of a Yin shortage, whereas if it is fast, it could be because of a Yang excess. Pulse rates within the usual range indicate good health.

• The pulse's rhythm describes how consistently (or inconsistently) it beats. Pulses can be normal, irregular, or intermittent according to traditional Chinese medicine.

A healthy person has a steady, regular pulse, while one that fluctuates or stops and starts may be a sign of internal disharmony.

• The breadth of the pulse is the extent to which it can be felt between two fingers. Pulses might be wide, normal, or narrow in Traditional Chinese Medicine.

If your pulse is wide, you may be experiencing abundance, whereas if it is small, you may be experiencing a lack. A healthy pulse width is estimated to be between 30 and 50 milliseconds.

• How strongly the pulse is felt under the fingertips is a measure of its strength. Strong, moderate, and weak pulses all exist in traditional Chinese medicine. If your pulse is strong, you may be in a state of abundance, whereas if it is weak, you may be deficient. around most cases, a healthy pulse rate is somewhere around the middle.

Pulse diagnosis in traditional Chinese medicine (TCM) is a very nuanced and sophisticated technique that calls for a great deal of training, experience, and clinical judgment.

Multiple aspects of the pulse are evaluated, and the TCM practitioner uses this information in conjunction with other diagnostic tools to arrive at a whole picture of the patient's health and make treatment decisions.

CHAPTER FOUR
Traditional Chinese Medicine Interpretations Of Various Pulse Characteristics

For practitioners of traditional Chinese medicine (TCM), interpreting one's pulse might provide information about the health of one's organs and meridians based on the quality of the pulse.

The Traditional Chinese Medicine (TCM) interpretations of several frequent pulse characteristics are as follows:

• A floating (superficial) pulse is one that is experienced on the skin's surface and does not go deep. It could have the sense of floating or be very compressible. Conditions of exterior or Yang excess, such fever, acute illness, or external pathogenic invasion, are related with this pulse quality.

• A deep, powerful pulse that can be felt much below the skin's surface is said to have a sinking (deep) pulse. It could feel like a deep, throbbing pulse. diseases of interior or Yin excess, such cold, chronic diseases, or internal organ disorders, are related with this pulse quality.

• A sluggish pulse is one that beats at a rate of 60 or less per minute. Conditions of cold or Yin deficiency, like cold syndromes, hypothyroidism, or vital energy insufficiency, are linked to this pulse quality.

• A rapid pulse is one that beats at a rate of more than ninety per minute. Fever, inflammation, hyperthyroidism, and an abundance of vital energy are all examples of conditions associated with an excess of heat or Yang.

• A regular pulse is one in which the beats occur at uniform intervals. This type of pulse is normal and represents a balanced physical state.

• An irregular heartbeat is characterized by beats that are spaced out at erratic intervals. Disharmony or imbalance in the body, such as an irregular heartbeat, arrhythmia, or stress, may be indicated by this characteristic of the pulse.

• One with a wide or thick pulse has a strong and complete quality. Conditions characterized by fullness or inflammation, high blood pressure, or fluid retention are linked to this type of pulse quality.

• A faint and hollow quality is indicated by a thin pulse, so named because of the short breadth of the pulse. Conditions of deficiency or emptiness, such as low vitality, low blood volume, or poor circulation, are linked to this type of pulse quality.

• A strong pulse is one that is brisk and jarring, suggesting an abundance of energy. Conditions of inflammation, high heat, or an excess of bodily fluids are all related with this type of pulse quality.

• A weak pulse is one that lacks strength and vitality and indicates an energy deficit. Deficiencies in vital energy, blood, or circulation are all conditions associated with this pulse quality.

To fully grasp a patient's health situation, a TCM practitioner must evaluate different pulse characteristics in addition to other diagnostic tools.

To get at an accurate diagnosis and appropriate treatment plan, a TCM practitioner will take into account a number of aspects, one of which is the context in which the patient's pulse characteristics are being interpreted.

Pattern And Imbalance Detection Through Pulse Analysis

Traditional Chinese medicine (TCM) relies on pulse diagnosis, which involves the careful observation and interpretation of numerous aspects of the pulse, to uncover patterns and imbalances in the body. Here are some typical imbalances and patterns that can be detected by taking a patient's pulse:

• In Traditional Chinese Medicine, the body is seen as a living system comprised of opposing energies known as Yin and Yang. Pulse diagnostic is a useful tool for detecting a Yin-Yang imbalance.

An outer pattern with Yang excess may be indicated by a pulse that floats weakly and lacks depth, whereas an inner pattern with Yin excess may be indicated by a pulse that sinks forcefully.

• Insufficiency and excess are both detectable by pulse analysis. An excess of heat or Yang energy, for instance, can be detected by a rapid but weak pulse, whereas a rapid but strong and forceful pulse may suggest a deficit of Qi (vital energy).

• Disharmony in the organs, according to TCM theory, which holds that each organ has its unique pulse position and quality. A practitioner of traditional Chinese medicine (TCM) can evaluate the health of your internal organs by palpating your pulse at several locations.

A strong and forceful pulse at the Liver position may suggest Liver Qi stagnation, whereas a weak and thin pulse at the Kidney position may indicate Kidney Qi deficiency.

• In TCM, organs and meridians are divided into five groups, each of which corresponds to one of the five elements (Water, Wood, Fire, Earth, and Metal). A quick heartbeat, on the other hand, may be indicative of a Fire element imbalance, while a wiry pulse may indicate a Wood element deficiency.

- Pulse diagnostics can tell the difference between illnesses that originate on the inside and those that come from the outside. When the pulse is light and airy, it may indicate an exterior pathogenic invasion (such as from cold or wind), but when it is deep and strong, it may indicate a problem of an internal organ (such as from excess heat).

- Emotional and stress-related factors: According to traditional Chinese medicine, these factors can alter the body's energy flow and pulse characteristics. An irregular or choppy pulse, for example, may suggest emotional stress or anxiety, and can be detected using pulse diagnostic.

• Constitutional factors: When evaluating a patient's health, TCM takes into account a person's unique set of characteristics, including their constitution.

A constitutional Qi shortage, as indicated by a weak pulse, or a strong, forceful pulse, as indicated by a healthy constitution, can be revealed by pulse diagnosis.

Pulse diagnosis in Traditional Chinese Medicine (TCM) is a personalized diagnostic procedure that calls for a great deal of talent and experience to achieve.

To arrive at a correct diagnosis and treatment strategy, it should be utilized in tandem with other TCM diagnostic procedures and a complete picture of the patient's health.

CHAPTER FIVE
Classifying Pulse Results As Either Excess Or Deficient

Traditional Chinese medicine (TCM) relies on pulse diagnosis, which involves the careful observation and interpretation of numerous aspects of the pulse to distinguish between excess and deficiency states. Here are some broad principles for using pulse results to distinguish between excess and deficiency states:

1. When the pulse has an excessive or excessive-sounding quality, we call it an excess condition. Some characteristics of the pulse that can indicate an overabundance of anything else are:

• Strong, full, and forceful pulses may be an indicator of an excess condition, such as an overabundance of Qi or blood.

• Excessive conditions, such high body temperature or an acute disease, may be reflected in a pulse that is quick or rapid.

• An overabundance of phlegm or moisture, for example, can be indicated by a wide or broad pulse.

• Slippery: An overabundance of moisture or pathogenic elements may be the cause of a smooth pulse.

2. Deficiency states are characterized by a lack of, or a lack of strength in, the pulse. Some indicators of deficient states in the pulse are:

• Deficiencies in Qi, blood, or Yin might manifest as a weak pulse, thus it is important to keep an eye out for these symptoms.

• A thin or tiny pulse may be an indicator of a deficiency, such as low blood or fluid levels.

• A slow or sluggish pulse may be an indication of a deficiency, such as a lack of Yang or a persistent disease.

• An empty or hollow pulse may be an indication of a deficiency, such as a lack of Qi or Yin.

Pulse diagnosis in Traditional Chinese Medicine is a highly

nuanced and sophisticated art that calls for the acute observation and interpretation of a wide variety of pulse properties at a variety of pulse locations.

In order to accurately distinguish between excess and deficient problems, the TCM practitioner will also take into account other clinical data, such as the patient's health history, symptoms, tongue diagnosis, and other diagnostic methods. The key to effective treatment that addresses the patient's unique needs is a correct diagnosis.

Heart And Circulatory System Diagnostics By Pulse

The Heart location pulse is taken from the radial artery on the radial side of the tendon of the flexor carpi radialis at the distal wrist to evaluate cardiovascular health in traditional Chinese medicine (TCM).

Pulse characteristics at the Heart location can reveal details about the condition of the heart's Qi and blood, as well as the cardiovascular system as a whole.

Pulse diagnostic for the TCM heart and cardiovascular system includes the following examples:

• Insufficient Qi in the Heart can manifest as a weak or soft pulse when palpated at the Heart position.

This could be the result of a depleted Heart Qi brought on by factors like prolonged illness, extreme stress, or exhaustion. Fatigue, heart palpitations, and shortness of breath are some of the possible additional symptoms.

• A weak or very tiny pulse in the chest region may be an indication of a lack of blood supply to the heart. Possible causes include the Heart's inability to produce enough blood due to factors including chronic disease, poor diet, or blood loss. Pale skin, lightheadedness, and memory loss are among possible side effects.

• Excessive heat in the Heart, or Heart fire, can manifest as a quick, powerful pulse at the Heart position. Stress, anxiety, or eating too many fatty or spicy meals could be to blame. Insomnia, flushing, and agitation are some of the other possible side effects.

• A lack of fullness in the Heart pulse may be a sign of Heart Yin deficit. A lack of Yin, the body's cooling and nourishing feature, could be to blame for this.

Yin deficit can occur as a result of chronic sickness, age, or eating too many spicy or acidic foods. Night sweats, hot flashes, and irritability may also occur.

• Stagnation of the blood supply to the heart might manifest as an irregular or erratic heartbeat. Trauma, blood clots, and other circulatory problems can cause blockages or stagnation in the Heart or blood arteries, leading to these symptoms. Chest discomfort, palpitations, and cyanosis are some of the possible further symptoms.

For an appropriate assessment of the Heart and circulatory system, it is crucial to highlight that TCM pulse diagnosis is a complicated and nuanced procedure that necessitates much training and experience.

The TCM practitioner will take the patient's pulse qualities into account alongside other clinical findings like the patient's health history, symptoms, tongue diagnosis, and other diagnostic methods to make an accurate diagnosis and formulate an effective treatment plan. For proper diagnosis and treatment, it is recommended that you see a trained TCM professional.

Pulse Analysis For Respiratory And Pulmonary Conditions

The Lung position pulse is taken from the radial artery at the distal wrist, on the radial side of the tendon of the flexor carpi radialis, and is used to evaluate the health of the lungs and respiratory system in accordance with traditional Chinese medicine (TCM).

The Lung position's pulse properties can reveal a lot about the respiratory system's health, including how your Lung Qi, Yin, and Yang are doing.

Examples of Pulse Diagnosis in Traditional Chinese Medicine for the Lungs and Respiratory System

• When the pulse is weak or absent in the Lung location, this may be a sign of Lung Qi shortage. The Lung Qi may be depleted owing to reasons such as long-term disease, poor diet, or the surrounding environment. Frequent respiratory infections, a weak voice, and shortness of breath may also be present.

• Deficiency of Lung Yin might be indicated by a pulse that is absent or floats in the Lung location. Chronic disease, dryness, or eating too many spicy and energizing foods can all lead to a Yin deficiency, which can have this effect. Night sweats, a dry cough, and a dry throat may also be present.

• Excessive heat in the lungs, or Lung heat, might be indicated by a quick and powerful pulse at the Lung location. Environmental factors, inflammation, and acute or chronic respiratory infections are all possible causes. A sore throat, fever, and cough with yellow or green sputum may also be present.

• A slick or oily feeling on the pulse when placed at the Lung position could be an indication of mucus in the lungs. Poor diet, persistent respiratory infections, and impaired digestion can all contribute to an overabundance of phlegm.

There may also be other symptoms like as a productive cough, chest congestion, and shortness of breath.

• A choppy or irregular pulse in the Lung area may be a sign of qi stasis in the Lung. This could be the result of mental stress, breathing problems, or some other obstruction or stagnation of Qi flow in the Lungs. Tightness in the chest, sighing, and erratic emotions may also be present.

When assessing the health of the lungs and respiratory system, TCM practitioners rely heavily on pulse diagnosis, which is a sophisticated and nuanced procedure that necessitates extensive training and expertise.

The TCM practitioner will take the patient's pulse qualities into account alongside other clinical findings like the patient's health history, symptoms, tongue diagnosis, and other diagnostic methods to make an accurate diagnosis and formulate an effective treatment plan. For proper diagnosis and treatment, it is recommended that you see a trained TCM professional.

CHAPTER SIX
Liver And Gallbladder Diagnosis Using Pulse Examination

In traditional Chinese medicine (TCM), the health of the Liver and Gallbladder are evaluated by taking the pulse at the Liver and Gallbladder positions, respectively located on the radial artery at the distal wrist on the radial side of the tendon of the flexor carpi radialis and the tendon of the flexor carpi ulnaris.

Examples of Liver and Gallbladder Pulse Diagnosis in Traditional Chinese Medicine

• A stringy or wiry pulse in the Liver area may be a sign of Liver Qi stagnation. This can happen when the Liver Qi is blocked, which can happen when there is emotional tension, frustration, or unresolved emotions. Abdominal distension or pain, impatience, and mood swings are also possible side effects.

• A lack of thick, strong pulse at the Liver location may be a sign of Liver Blood insufficiency. Causes of blood shortage include long-term illness, malnutrition, and heavy bleeding. Tiredness, a whitish complexion, and lightheadedness may also be present.

• Excessive heat in the Liver, also known as Liver Fire, might be indicated by a quick and powerful pulse in the Liver location. Possible causes include mental strain, inflammation, or eating too many spicy foods. Angry outbursts, impatience, bloodshot eyes, and a parched tongue are possible side effects.

• Gallbladder Dampness: A slick or oily feeling on the pulse at the gallbladder region could be a sign of gallbladder dampness. Possible causes include gallbladder dysfunction owing to dietary deficiencies or intestinal problems. Some people also experience nausea, loss of appetite, and a heaviness in the chest or belly.

• Weak or absent pulse at the gallbladder site may indicate a Qi shortage in the gallbladder. This could be the outcome of a depleted Gallbladder Qi brought on by, among other things, long-term disease or bad diet. Digestion problems like bloating, belching, and gas may also present themselves.

To properly evaluate the health of the Liver, Gallbladder, and related meridian channels and functions, a practitioner of Traditional Chinese Medicine (TCM) must have extensive training and expertise with the art of pulse diagnosis.

The TCM practitioner will take the patient's pulse qualities into account alongside other clinical findings like the patient's health history, symptoms, tongue diagnosis, and other diagnostic methods to make an accurate diagnosis and formulate an effective treatment plan. For proper diagnosis and treatment, it is recommended that you see a trained TCM professional.

Spleen And Digestive System Pulse Analysis

The Spleen position pulse, located on the medial side of the tendon of the flexor carpi radialis at the distal wrist, is used to evaluate the health of the Spleen and the digestive system as a whole in traditional Chinese medicine (TCM).

Traditional Chinese Medicine (TCM) pulse diagnosis examples for the Spleen and digestive system:

• Weak or absent pulse at the Spleen position may be an indication of a Qi shortage in the Spleen. This could be the result of a deficiency in Spleen Qi brought on by things like an unhealthy diet, poor digestion, long-term illness, or any other issue. Fatigue, loss of appetite, diarrhea, and stomach bloating are some of the other symptoms that may occur.

• Dampness in the spleen can be detected by feeling a slippery or greasy pulse at the spleen site. The Spleen may be malfunctioning as a result of unhealthy eating habits or excessive weight gain. Weight gain, nausea, loss of appetite, and a greasy film on the tongue are also possible symptoms.

• A sluggish or weak pulse in the Spleen position may be an indication of a Yang deficiency in the Spleen. Possible causes include a depleted Spleen Yang brought on by long-term illness, extreme cold, or some other circumstance. Chills, weakness, loss of appetite, diarrhea, and stomach bloating are some of the other symptoms that may occur.

• A lack of or weak pulse in the Spleen position may suggest a lack of or weak pulse in the Spleen. Possible causes include prolonged disease, insufficient nutrition, or something else that leads to a lack of Blood. Weakness, pallor, a lack of appetite, and diarrhoea may also be present.

• Food stagnation might be indicated by a choppy or uneven pulse in the Spleen location. This can happen when undigested food builds up in the digestive track for various reasons, including a poor diet, overeating, or both. Abdominal swelling, burping, and noxious gas may also accompany this condition.

To effectively assess the status of the Spleen, the digestive system, and their related meridians and functions, it is vital to recognize that pulse diagnosis in TCM is a complicated and nuanced procedure that takes much training and expertise.

The TCM practitioner will take the patient's pulse qualities into account alongside other clinical findings like the patient's health history, symptoms, tongue diagnosis, and other diagnostic methods to make an accurate diagnosis and formulate an effective treatment plan.

For proper diagnosis and treatment, it is recommended that you see a trained TCM professional.

Kidney And Urinary System Diagnosis By Pulse Analysis

The Kidney position pulse is taken on the lateral side of the tendon of the flexor carpi ulnaris at the distal wrist to evaluate the health of the urinary system and the Kidneys in accordance with traditional Chinese medicine (TCM).

Some examples of TCM kidney and urine system pulse diagnostic are as follows:

• An indicator of Kidney Yin shortage is a thin, weak, or floaty pulse in the Kidney position. This could be the result of low Yin levels brought on by things like prolonged illness or overexposure to heat. Night sweats, hot flashes, dry mouth, dry throat, and a red tongue with little or no coating are sometimes present as well.

• Kidney Yang Deficiency: Symptoms include a weak, slow, or deep pulse when palpating the Kidney area.

The Kidney Yang may have been depleted owing to long-term disease, extreme cold, or some other circumstance.

A pale or swollen tongue, extreme weakness, frequent urination, low back discomfort, and icy extremities are all possible.

• Weak or absent pulse at the Kidney location may indicate a Qi shortage in the Kidneys. Possible causes include a deficiency in Kidney Qi brought on by long-term disease or poor diet. Fatigue, weakness, increased urination, lower back pain, and a pale or swollen tongue may also be present.

• Lack of Jing in the Kidneys can manifest as a weak or absent pulse when palpating that area of the body. Jing, the essence of life and vigor in TCM, can be depleted by things like genetics and constitution, long-term disease, and overwork.

Paleness or swelling of the tongue may also occur, and other symptoms may include lethargy, weakness, stunted growth, infertility, and weariness.

• The presence of a wiry or choppy pulse in the Kidney position may be an indication of Qi stagnation in the Kidneys or urinary system.

This could be the result of mental or emotional strain, bad habits, or some other impediment to the free passage of Qi in the Kidneys.

Emotional symptoms like anxiety or anger may also occur alongside physical symptoms like urine frequency, urgency, or trouble urinating.

To properly evaluate the condition of the Kidneys, urinary system, and associated meridian channels and bodily processes through pulse diagnosis in TCM, one must have extensive training and expertise.

The TCM practitioner will take the patient's pulse qualities into account alongside other clinical findings like the patient's health history, symptoms, tongue diagnosis, and other diagnostic methods to make an accurate diagnosis and formulate an effective treatment plan. For proper diagnosis and treatment, it is recommended that you see a trained TCM professional.

CHAPTER SEVEN
Detecting Fertility Issues Through The Pulse

The uterus and ovaries in females and the prostate gland in males can both be evaluated using pulse diagnostic in traditional Chinese medicine (TCM). For TCM pulse diagnostics of the reproductive system, the following examples of pulse qualities and their interpretations are provided:

• The stagnation of blood in the reproductive system might manifest as a choppy or irregular pulse, especially at the Cun (middle) location. Hormonal disruptions, menstrual abnormalities, and other gynecological and urological disorders may contribute to this. Abdominal pain, unpleasant or heavy periods, blood clots during menstruation, and difficulties in sexual functioning may also be present.

• Stagnation of Qi in the reproductive system can manifest as a wiry or stiff pulse, especially in the Guan (proximal) position. This could be caused by factors that restrict the passage of Qi to the reproductive organs, such as emotional stress or unhealthy habits. Mood swings, irritability, bloating, and distention in the lower belly are sometimes present as well.

• Male and female reproductive health can be negatively impacted by a lack of Kidney Jing, which can be indicated by a thin or weak pulse.

According to TCM, kidney jing shortage can be caused by factors including genetics or constitution, long-term disease, or undue strain on the body. It is also possible to have exhaustion, weakness, infertility, a low libido, or a dysfunctional sexual life.

• A slippery or sloppy pulse may be an indication of phlegm or moisture buildup in the reproductive system.

Causes for this include insufficient nutrition, an overabundance of phlegm or dampness in the body, or problems with the reproductive system. Bloating, vaginal discharge, and urinary symptoms including frequent urination or hazy urine may also be present.

5. Discordant Yin and Yang Qualities in the Pulse May Indicate a Problem in the Reproductive System.

Yin deficiency may manifest as a weak or slow pulse, whereas Yang excess may manifest as a rapid or powerful pulse. Hormonal fluctuations, bad behaviors, and medical problems that influence the reproductive system can all contribute to this kind of discord.

Pulse diagnosis in Traditional Chinese Medicine (TCM) is a sophisticated and subtle procedure that necessitates extensive knowledge and expertise to correctly evaluate the reproductive system and formulate an effective treatment plan.

In order to make an accurate diagnosis and formulate a personalized treatment plan, the TCM practitioner will take into account the pulse qualities in addition to other clinical data such as the patient's medical history, symptoms, tongue diagnosis, and other diagnostic procedures.

If you are experiencing symptoms related to your reproductive system, it is important to see a trained TCM practitioner for an appropriate diagnosis and treatment plan.

Musculoskeletal System Pulse Analysis

Traditional Chinese medicine (TCM) practitioners employ pulse diagnosis to evaluate the health of their patients' musculoskeletal structures.

Here are some instances of musculoskeletal-related pulse characteristics and their interpretations in traditional Chinese medicine:

• Indicators of localized blood or Qi stagnation include a choppy or irregular pulse, especially at the pulse point corresponding to the affected portion of the musculoskeletal system.

Possible causes include inflammation in the musculoskeletal system, as well as trauma, injury, and overuse. Pain, edema, decreased range of motion, and/or stiffness in the affected area may also be present.

• Stagnation of the Qi in the musculoskeletal system is indicated by a wiry or tense pulse, especially in the Guan (proximal) position. The entire flow of Qi in the musculoskeletal system may be disrupted due to factors including poor circulation, inactivity, or chronic stress. Muscle tension, muscle spasms, and generalized body aches and pains are sometimes present as well.

• Deficiency: A weak or thin pulse may be an indication of a Yin or Yang deficiency in the musculoskeletal system. In TCM, deficiency is commonly associated with circumstances that diminish the body's resources, such as inadequate nutrition, lack of rest, or chronic sickness. Weakness, weariness, low muscular tone, and a prolonged recovery from traumas may also be present.

• An accumulation of dampness or phlegm in the musculoskeletal system might manifest as a slippery or soggy pulse. This could be the result of dietary deficiencies, too much phlegm, or some other issue affecting the musculoskeletal system. Additional signs may include localized swelling, heaviness, or a fullness sensation.

5. Invasion of the wind into the musculoskeletal system might manifest as a floating or shifting pulse. According to TCM, wind is one of the external infections that can invade the body and create transient and dispersive symptoms

including muscular spasms, twitches, and joint discomfort.

Sensitivity to climate change and fluctuation of symptoms in response to physical exercise may also be present.

In Traditional Chinese Medicine (TCM), pulse diagnosis is a complicated and nuanced procedure used to analyze the health of the musculoskeletal system and choose the best course of therapy.

In order to make an accurate diagnosis and formulate a personalized treatment plan, the TCM practitioner will take into account the pulse qualities in addition to other clinical data such as the patient's medical history, symptoms, tongue diagnosis, and other diagnostic procedures. If you are experiencing pain in your muscles or bones, it is best to see a trained TCM professional for an accurate diagnosis and effective treatment.

CHAPTER EIGHT
Integrating Pulse Analysis With Traditional Chinese Medicine Techniques

Pulse diagnosis is used in conjunction with other diagnostic tools in TCM to help practitioners get a full picture of the patient's health. Some ways in which pulse analysis can complement other TCM diagnostic techniques are given below.

• The tongue is used in diagnosis because it is thought to reflect the health of the patient's internal organs. Along with pulse diagnosis, a practitioner of traditional Chinese medicine (TCM) can learn about a patient's overall health by observing the tongue's color, coating, wetness, and other characteristics.

• Acupuncture point palpation is another diagnostic tool used by TCM practitioners in addition to taking the patient's pulse. A patient's health status and prospective treatments can be further understood by the identification of tender or sensitive points, which may indicate an imbalance or blockage in the flow of Qi in a particular meridian.

• An in-depth patient interview and history are essential to a correct

TCM diagnosis. In order to get a full picture of the patient's health, the practitioner may ask questions regarding the patient's medical history, lifestyle, diet, sleep patterns, emotional state, and other factors. Findings from taking the pulse can be correlated with this data to reveal patterns and imbalances inside the body.

• TCM practitioners pay close attention to the patient's skin tone, eyes, nails, and general demeanor as part of their diagnostic process. When paired with pulse diagnostics, these findings can provide invaluable insight into the patient's internal health, allowing for more precise diagnosis and treatment.

• Pulse diagnosis is frequently employed in tandem with pattern differentiation, the process of determining underlying causes of a patient's health problems by analyzing their constellation of symptoms, indicators, and diagnostic findings. Understanding the nature of the pattern, such as excess or deficiency, through pulse diagnosis can aid in the selection of effective TCM treatment methods.

A more complete picture of the patient's health situation, patterns of disharmony, and an individualized treatment plan for restoring balance and promoting health can be attained when pulse diagnosis is used in conjunction with other TCM diagnostic procedures. If you want to get the most out of your TCM therapy, it is best to see a practitioner who is well-versed in a variety of diagnostic techniques.

Taking A Patient's Pulse To Diagnose Serious Or Ongoing Health Issues

Traditional Chinese medicine (TCM) pulse diagnostic can be utilized for both acute and chronic illnesses. A chronic condition is one that lasts for an extended period of time, while a complex condition may involve several different organs or systems that all interact with one another.

Conditions like these often have underlying imbalances and patterns of disharmony, and pulse diagnostics can shed light on these.

Traditional Chinese medicine (TCM) practitioners may use a variety of methods, including:

• To detect even the most minute variations in the pulse's quality, a TCM practitioner may conduct a more in-depth examination.

In order to get a full picture of the patient's health, it may be necessary to palpate multiple pulse locations on both wrists with changing pressures and evaluate the pulse's depth, rate, rhythm, width, strength, and other features.

• Excess or deficiency patterns, as well as patterns associated to the organs or systems involved in the complex or chronic illness, can be identified using pulse diagnostics.

By recognizing these trends, TCM doctors may create individualized treatment plans that go to the bottom of what is wrong and help bring the body back into harmony.

• Combining Pulse Diagnosis with Other Traditional Chinese Medicine Diagnostic Techniques To obtain a more thorough assessment of the patient's health condition, pulse diagnosis can be combined with other TCM diagnostic techniques, such as tongue diagnosis, palpation of acupuncture points, history taking, patient interview, and observation of physical appearance.

This can aid in determining the most effective course of treatment for the complex or chronic ailment by illuminating underlying imbalances and trends.

• Pulse diagnosis can be used to monitor the progression of complex and chronic illnesses over time by recording any changes in the quality of the pulse.

This can aid in monitoring the patient's state and the treatment plan's efficacy, allowing for course correction if necessary.

• Customized Care Traditional Chinese Medicine (TCM) frequently employs tailored care plans when treating complex and chronic diseases. By taking into account the patient's constitution, any underlying imbalances, and any other factors that may be contributing to the ailment, TCM practitioners can tailor the treatment strategy based on the unique pulse findings of each patient.

When it comes to complex and chronic diseases, TCM practitioners often turn to pulse diagnosis to get insight into the underlying imbalances and patterns of disharmony in the body. However, for an appropriate assessment and individualized treatment plan, it is vital to visit a skilled TCM practitioner who has experience utilizing pulse diagnosis and other diagnostic procedures for complex and chronic diseases.

CHAPTER NINE
Identifying Psychological And Emotional Disorders By Taking A Patient's Pulse

Emotional and mental health abnormalities can also be diagnosed using pulse diagnostic in TCM. Pulse quality can be an indicator of emotional and psychological abnormalities, which are central to TCM's understanding of health and wellness.

The following are some of the factors that TCM doctors may take into account when employing pulse diagnosis to treat mental and emotional disorders:

• Assessing the depth, pace, rhythm, width, and intensity of the pulse can help traditional Chinese medicine (TCM) practitioners diagnose emotional or psychological problems.

A fast or wiry pulse, for instance, may be indicative of intense emotions like wrath or impatience, whereas a slow or weak pulse may indicate emotional weakness or stagnation.

• When diagnosing emotional or psychological abnormalities, TCM practitioners may also look for telltale signs in the patient's pulse.

Anxiety and worry may be connected with a floating pulse (a pulse that feels like it is floating on the surface), whereas emotional instability and mood swings may be associated with a slippery pulse (a pulse that feels smooth and sliding).

• Certain patterns of disharmony related to emotional or psychological abnormalities can be identified by TCM practitioners.

These patterns include liver qi stagnation, heart fire, spleen deficiency, and kidney deficiency. These regularities may shed light on physical imbalances that are at the root of the emotional or psychological distress.

• You can get a more complete picture of the patient's emotional and psychological imbalances by integrating pulse diagnosis with other TCM diagnostic methods like tongue diagnosis, palpation of acupuncture points, patient interview, and observation of physical and emotional symptoms. This information can be used as a reference when deciding on a course of treatment.

• Emotional and psychological disorders in TCM need an

individualized treatment plan just like any other condition. Each patient's constitution, underlying imbalances, and emotional and psychological state are unique, and so is the treatment plan that TCM practitioners can create using pulse diagnosis.

TCM practitioners can use pulse diagnosis to get insight into the root causes of emotional and psychological discord by revealing patterns of disharmony in the body.

However, for an appropriate assessment and individualized treatment plan, it is essential to visit a skilled TCM practitioner who has experience utilizing pulse diagnosis and other diagnostic procedures for emotional and psychological imbalances.

Herbal medicine, acupuncture, dietary and lifestyle suggestions, and other TCM techniques may all play a role in treating emotional and psychological disorders, depending on the patient's specific needs.

Diagnosis Via The Pulse For Children And Other Vulnerable Groups

Traditional Chinese medicine (TCM) pulse diagnosis can be utilized with children and other special groups, albeit it may need to be adapted slightly to account for their specific traits and health situations. Some things to think about are as follows:

• During pulse diagnosis, small toddlers and infants may not be as cooperative or able to articulate their feelings as older patients. More observation, intuition, and probing of less common spots like the fontanelles and abdomen may be required of TCM practitioners. When taking the pulse of a child, it is vital to take your time, be patient, and use approaches that are age and developmentally appropriate.

• Since children's bodies are still maturing and changing, the properties of their pulses may vary from those of adults. Changes in the pace, rhythm, width, strength, and depth of the pulse may be used by TCM practitioners as indicators of health.

For instance, a constitutional or developmental issue can be indicated by a sluggish or deep pulse, while a quick or weak pulse in a child might signal an acute disease.

• Because of their rapid growth and development, pediatric patients' pulses may fluctuate over time.

Traditional Chinese Medicine (TCM) practitioners may need to evaluate the child's pulse in light of their age and stage of development. The pulse of a young child may be quick and shallow, while that of a teenager may be slower and deeper.

• Children's Pulses might be affected by their own constitutional variables. When assessing a child's pulse quality and general health, TCM practitioners may think about the child's constitutional type, such as whether they are more yin or yang.

One youngster may have a stronger and more forceful pulse because of their yang constitution, whereas another child with a yin constitution may have a weaker and more delicate pulse.

• Additionally, pregnant women, the elderly, and those with chronic health concerns can also benefit from a pulse diagnostic. When interpreting the pulses of these populations, TCM doctors may need to account for unique physiological changes or clinical issues.

In pregnant women, for instance, the pulse may be altered by hormonal changes and increased blood volume, while in the elderly, alterations to the circulatory system may cause the pulse to be weaker and more erratic.

• As with other populations, TCM diagnostic methods such as tongue diagnosis, palpation of acupuncture points, patient interview, and observation of physical and emotional symptoms can be integrated with pulse diagnosis for pediatric patients and special populations to obtain a more thorough evaluation. When working with underserved communities, TCM practitioners may also take into account Western medical diagnosis and treatment strategies.

• It is essential to ensure the comfort and cooperation of pediatric patients and other special populations by maintaining open lines of communication throughout the pulse diagnostic process.

TCM doctors should take into account the safety and preferences of vulnerable populations, such as pregnant women and the elderly, and tailor their explanations of the treatment procedure to each patient's age group.

When used by trained practitioners, TCM pulse diagnosis can shed light on the health of children and other vulnerable populations, allowing for more informed treatment decisions.

If you want an accurate diagnosis and individualized treatment plans that take into account these groups' particular traits and health concerns, you need to see a trained TCM practitioner who has expertise working with them.

CHAPTER TEN
Integrating Pulse Analysis With Traditional Chinese Medicine

Traditional Chinese medicine (TCM) treatment plans often include pulse diagnosis as an integral part of the diagnostic process.

• Information gleaned through pulse diagnosis, such as pulse characteristics, rhythms, and imbalances, can aid TCM practitioners in developing patient-specific treatment plans. For instance, if the diagnosis of the patient's pulse reveals an excess pattern with a quick and powerful pulse, the treatment plan may center on removing excess and minimizing excessive energy or stagnation.

However, if a weak and slow pulse suggests a deficiency pattern, the treatment may center on nourishing and tonifying the body to improve the weak organs or systems.

• Pulse diagnosis can also be used to track how well a patient responds to treatment over time. During following therapy sessions, TCM practitioners may re-evaluate the pulse to see if the properties of the pulse have improved or altered, indicating good changes in the patient's health. Changes in pulse characteristics can inform course corrections for better therapeutic results.

• Using a pulse diagnostic, practitioners of traditional Chinese medicine (TCM) can better determine which treatment methods will be most effective.

Practitioners of traditional Chinese medicine (TCM) may use the results of a pulse diagnosis to determine the most effective combination of acupuncture sites, herbal formulae, dietary advice, lifestyle modifications, and other TCM interventions to correct the underlying imbalances and patterns seen in the patient's pulse.

To eliminate heat from the body, for instance, acupuncture points and herbal formulae with cooling characteristics may be chosen by TCM practitioners if a pulse diagnosis reveals a heat pattern.

• Pulse diagnosis can aid TCM doctors in determining the root of a patient's health problems. TCM practitioners can learn about the underlying causes of a patient's ailment, such as emotional imbalances, lifestyle variables, dietary habits, or external influences, by observing the quality and patterns of the patient's pulse.

This knowledge can help shape a treatment strategy that gets to the bottom of the patient's health problems, not just the symptoms.

• Pulse diagnosis in TCM also has the added benefit of strengthening the practitioner-patient bond. Patients may have a more invested and empowering experience with their healthcare when they are actively involved in the diagnosis process, such as through pulse palpation.

Practitioners of traditional Chinese medicine (TCM) can also employ pulse diagnosis as a teaching tool, providing patients with information about their diagnoses and treatment plans.

By incorporating pulse diagnosis into TCM treatment plans, practitioners can learn more about their patients' health conditions, create personalized plans of care, track their patients' progress, choose the most effective TCM modalities, pinpoint the root of their symptoms, and build stronger relationships with their patients. If you want an accurate diagnosis and individualized treatment programs that take into account your specific needs and health situations, you should see a trained TCM practitioner who specializes in pulse diagnostics.

Learning To Palpate

Traditional Chinese medicine (TCM) pulse diagnosis is a discipline that involves talent, experience, and an in-depth understanding of TCM concepts and ideas.

Here are some suggestions to hone your palpation abilities for identifying pulses:

• Start by learning the theories and principles behind TCM pulse diagnosis through your own study. Read TCM literature, go to lectures or seminars, and take lessons from seasoned TCM professionals to gain an understanding of pulse characteristics, patterns, and imbalances.

• Spend a lot of time watching and practicing pulse palpation. Learn about pulse diagnosis by first seeing skilled TCM doctors at work. You should observe their hand placement, pressure, and technique carefully.

The next step is to hone your tactile sensitivity and discriminating skills by practicing on a range of patients with varying pulse quality, patterns, and imbalances.

• Pulse diagnosis relies heavily on the correct posture of the hands. Accurately palpating the various pulse characteristics and patterns requires precise finger positioning on the radial artery. To get a good read on the pulse's properties including depth, pace, rhythm, width, and strength, try out a few various hand placements to see what works best for you.

• The ability to feel the pulse's subtleties requires the development of tactile sensitivity. Apply steady, light pressure with your fingertips on the radial artery, taking care not to obstruct the patient's pulse or cause unnecessary pain. Paying attention to the varied properties of the pulse beneath your fingertips is a great way to train your sense of touch.

• Learn to Identify Variations in Pulse Quality Exercise your palpation skills by learning to identify variations in pulse quality, patterns, and imbalances.

Learn to recognize the difference between a sluggish pulse and a quick pulse, a weak pulse and a powerful one, a floating pulse and a deep one, a slick pulse and a wiry one, and so on. Learning to accurately recognize distinct pulse characteristics requires practice and the guidance of seasoned professionals.

• Pulse diagnosis relies heavily on the practitioner's ability to exercise clinical judgment. It entails combining the results of pulse palpation with those of other TCM diagnostic tools, including as tongue diagnosis, patient history, symptoms, and other examination findings, to generate a whole picture of the patient's health status. Your ability to exercise clinical judgment and make sound decisions in the clinic will improve with time and experience.

• You can improve your palpation abilities by regularly seeking comments and coaching from seasoned TCM practitioners.

Inquire about the hand placement, pressure, and technique you are using. You can learn more about the various pulse patterns and imbalances by talking about specific instances with seasoned practitioners.

• Regular practice is essential for developing skilled palpation. Your ability to recognize variations in pulse quality, pattern, and imbalance will improve with experience. Gain useful experience by working with a wide range of patients of varying ages and ailments.

In order to become proficient in palpating the pulse, one must be patient, practice, and experience. In order to become proficient in pulse diagnosis in TCM, it is necessary to consistently learn, observe, practice, and seek help from experienced practitioners.

CHAPTER ELEVEN
Diagnostic Traps And Difficulties In Pulse Analysis

Traditional Chinese medicine (TCM) pulse diagnosis is a highly sophisticated diagnostic technique that calls for expert hands and a thorough familiarity with TCM tenets and theories. Practitioners may face a number of obstacles and difficulties when conducting a pulse diagnostic. Here are a few examples:

• Poor education and experience: Pulse diagnosis is a complex skill that requires significant time and effort to master. Inadequate training and experience can lead to incorrect diagnosis and ineffective treatment approaches by preventing a practitioner from accurately assessing the pulse's characteristics, patterns, and imbalances.

• Variability and subjectivity: Different doctors may arrive at different conclusions while analyzing a patient's pulse. Variability in the results may be introduced by factors such as the practitioner's physical state, mood, and level of experience, all of which can affect the perception and interpretation of pulse characteristics.

• Consistency in findings cannot be guaranteed because of the influence of patient characteristics such as age, physical condition, body position, and emotional state. A weak pulse, for instance, may be an age-related alteration rather than a sign of a deficiency in an aged patient.

• How cooperative and relaxed the patient is during pulse diagnosis might also have an impact on the reliability of the results. It can be difficult to get a good read on the patient's pulse if they are nervous, agitated, or on the move.

• Inadequate evaluation Pulse diagnosis requires analyzing a wide range of pulse characteristics, patterns, and imbalances.

An incorrect diagnosis or vital information missed may occur from a superficial or narrowly-focused assessment of the pulse's properties.

• Pulse diagnosis in Traditional Chinese Medicine necessitates placing the data within the context of TCM principles and beliefs, which may be at odds with the Western medical paradigm. Integrating the pulse data with other diagnostic tools and coming up with an appropriate TCM treatment plan can be difficult.

• Different TCM schools or lineages may use different methodologies and have different interpretations when it comes to pulse diagnosis because there is no standardized approach. This may cause discrepancies in the results and interpretations of pulse diagnostics.

• Some health disorders, especially chronic and complex ones, might present with a wide variety of pulse characteristics, patterns, and imbalances, making it difficult to make an accurate assessment and interpretation of the data.

• It may take multiple assessments and observations of the patient's pulse before the qualities, patterns, and imbalances can be determined, hence patience is a virtue when performing a pulse diagnosis. Lack of patience or haste in the procedure can lead to erroneous results.

• Finally, it is crucial to take into account ethical factors such patient confidentiality, informed permission, and cultural and personal views when doing pulse diagnosis.

TCM's pulse diagnosis is an effective diagnostic tool, but it is not without its own caveats and difficulties.

Overcoming these obstacles and effectively interpreting the pulse data in the context of TCM principles to produce an effective treatment plan for patients requires proper training, experience, and clinical judgment.

Improving The Quality Of Pulse Diagnosis

Several methods exist in traditional Chinese medicine (TCM) for improving the precision and dependability of pulse diagnosis. Some ways to enhance the precision and dependability of pulse diagnosis are outlined below.

• To get a full picture of the pulse's properties, it is important to conduct a thorough evaluation that takes into account all of its aspects, including depth, rate, rhythm, width, and strength.

• Consistency in Method: When taking a patient's pulse, be consistent with finger placement, palpation depth, pressure, and duration of evaluation. Consistency in method reduces room for error, leading to more trustworthy findings.

• Make sure the patient is calm, at ease, and in a good posture for taking their pulse. Keep tension, anxiety, and movement to a minimum, as they can all have a negative impact on the heart rate.

• Acquire and hone your palpation abilities with extensive practice and experience. Accuracy in pulse diagnosis can be dramatically increased with proper hands-on instruction and supervised practice.

• In order to interpret the results of a TCM pulse diagnosis in light of the patient's overall health, medical history, symptoms, and other diagnostic methods, you will need to utilize your best clinical judgment and critical thinking skills. Do not draw inferences based on the pulse results alone; instead, think of them in the context of the whole evaluation.

• Learn Constantly: Stay abreast of new developments in TCM pulse diagnosis research, literature, and instruction. Improve the accuracy and consistency of your pulse diagnosis by learning more about TCM theories, pulse characteristics, patterns, and imbalances.

• Seek feedback from seasoned professionals and review cases to zero in on skill gaps and develop your practice. Any inaccuracies or biases in pulse diagnosis can be uncovered and corrected by regular evaluation and feedback.

• Consistency and trustworthiness in evaluation and interpretation are best achieved by adhering to a systematic system or approach for pulse diagnosis. When there are numerous doctors working on a patient, this can be especially useful.

• Working together, using tongue diagnosis, questions, and

observations in addition to the results of a pulse analysis can yield a more complete and accurate diagnosis in traditional Chinese medicine.

• Maintaining patient confidentiality, giving informed consent, and respecting cultural and personal views are all examples of ethical principles in pulse diagnosis that should be followed to ensure professional integrity and trustworthiness.

By employing these methods, TCM doctors can improve the precision and consistency of pulse diagnosis, ultimately providing patients with more targeted and successful treatment.

Conclusion

Pulse diagnosis is an essential diagnostic procedure in traditional Chinese medicine (TCM), and it entails analyzing the patient's pulse to learn about their organ, system, and general health. Competence in palpation, sound clinical judgment, and familiarity with TCM tenets are all prerequisites.

TCM relies heavily on pulse diagnosis to assess health, locate sources of imbalance, and inform the creation of individualized treatment strategies.

It is especially helpful in detecting complex and chronic diseases, emotional and psychological imbalances, and in patients from underserved communities like children.

However, there are also disadvantages and difficulties associated with pulse diagnosis, including as subjectivity, variability, and the requirement for constant skill improvement and standardization.

In the field of pulse diagnostics, it is imperative that professionals always work with the utmost integrity and care for their patients.

TCM practitioners can improve the accuracy and reliability of pulse diagnosis and provide optimal care for their patients by incorporating pulse diagnosis with other TCM diagnostic methods, maintaining consistency in technique, continually learning and improving palpation skills, and collaborating with other practitioners.

THE END